TURMERIC:
HOW TO USE IT FOR
YOUR WELLNESS

Overcome Inflammation, Enemy of Your Body

_____

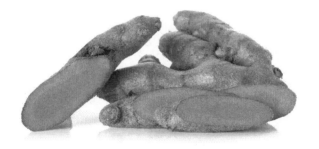

By Kathy Heshelow
Sublime Beauty Naturals® and Sublime Naturals

D1502872

[?]

Turmeric: How to Use It For Your Wellness. Overcome Inflammation, Enemy of Your Body. Part of the Sublime Wellness Lifestyle Series. Text copyright ® 2017 by Kathy Heshelow

ISBN: 9781521005378 ALL RIGHTS RESERVED

Published by Sublime Beauty Naturals®
11125 Park Blvd, Suite 104-103, Seminole FL 33772
ISBN 978-0-692-65198-8 (book)

Heshelow portrait by Heidi Haponowitz Photography

Printed in the United States

Disclaimer: This book and information is for reference and education, and represents my views and research, include the research and reference to clinical publications of others.

FDA Disclaimer

Preface

I was told by a doctor when I was a teenager that I would have a high chance ("almost probable", he said) of developing rheumatoid arthritis. I was an active and relatively athletic kid, and after looking up what the disease was, I decided I would take measures to try to never let it happen.

I learned that inflammation was the enemy.

So far (I am a baby-boomer who just turned 60), I have not developed rheumatoid arthritis, arthritis or any inflammatory disease. I have used turmeric for decades and I believe it is a strong reason why I have kept this disease at bay. I am a big fan of turmeric and boswellia (frankincense). I take a daily; have used curcumin (the active ingredient in turmeric) in cooking and recipes during the 16 years I lived in Paris, France and after. I follow an anti-inflammatory diet as much as possible.

When I formed a wellness-related company (Sublime Naturals), I knew that turmeric and anti-inflammatory products would be part of it along with products to help naturally support the immune system – and to share this with others. This short book is an outgrowth of these experiences, as is the new wellness lifestyle series of eBooks.

Reach out with any questions, and enjoy the short book!

Kathy Heshelow, founder
Sublime Beauty, Sublime Naturals, ZEN BOX,

Author of "Essential Oils Have Super Powers:
From Solving Everyday Wellness Problems to Taking on Superbugs"

"Secrets to a Better Immune System"

"Phytoceramides: Anti-Aging at its Best"

"The Crisis of Antibiotic-Resistant Bacteria – and How Essential Oils Help."

and many more...

Podcast: Essential Oil Zen
www.SublimeNaturals.com
www.Kathyheshelow.com

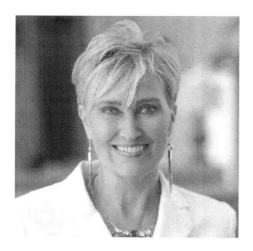

Table of Contents

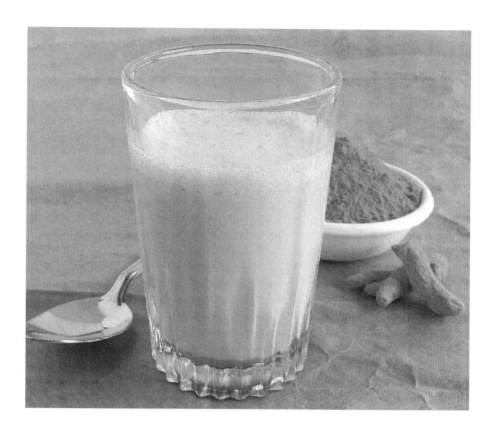

As a kid, whenever we got sick, my mom would take milk and put turmeric in it. That was our medicine. That was the cure-all. Some people turn to Robitussin.

- Aasif Mandvi

Chapter 1

WHY USE TURMERIC?
THE BENEFITS

Before we get into WHAT turmeric and curcumin (the active ingredient in turmeric) are, let's go over some of the benefits. It will help answer the question WHY use turmeric and why read this book.

There is excellent research and knowledge about turmeric showing clear health benefits. In fact, there are over 7,000 peer-reviewed studies on curcumin, the active ingredient in turmeric. There are over 1,000 scientific research papers on curcumin in PubMed. (a)

Turmeric has been actively used for centuries in India (it's in the curry spice!), China, Asian countries and Middle Eastern countries for many conditions and overall health, with good results. More "Western- style" clinical-medical studies have emerged to back up what people have known for a long time.

SOME OF THE BENEFITS ARE:

- IS ANTI-INFLAMMATORY

- FIGHTS AGAINST CANCER
- REDUCES STRESS

- BOOSTS THE IMMUNE SYSTEM
- IS A STRONG ANTIOXIDANT

- DECREASES HEART DISEASE RISK
  & SUPPORTS ARTERY HEALTH

- HELPS THE DIGESTIVE SYSTEM & CAN HELP PREVENT BOWEL CANCER

- HELPFUL FOR OILY SKIN, SENSITIVE SKIN, AGING SKIN & ECZEMA

- SUPPORTS HEALTHY BLOOD SUGAR LEVELS

- COULD HELP SLOW ALZHEIMER'S

& MORE...

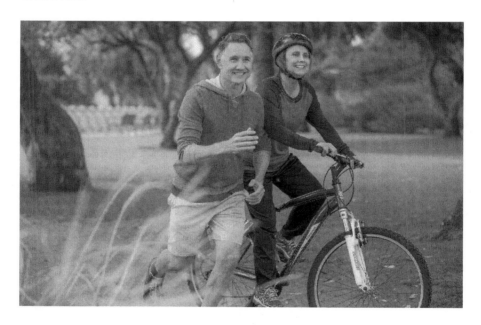

Turmeric is powerful for wellness. It is appropriate for all ages, on the FDA GRAS ("generally recognized as safe") list. Due to its special qualities (such as anti- inflammatory, possibly slowing Alzheimer's & supporting heart health), is especially helpful for the aging population.

BENEFITS – WHY USE TURMERIC

In Ayurvedic India, it has been used as an all-round tonic and internal cleanser for centuries. In Chinese medicine, it has been used for sores, bruises, chest pain, warming, tooth ache and was once a treatment for jaundice.

Recent studies in Japan have shown the relationship with interleukin (IL-6), which is the inflammatory cytokine involved in rheumatoid arthritis, and found that curcumin (the active component of turmeric) "significantly reduced" these inflammatory markers. (1)

Modern research has shown that regular ingestion of the spice may help prevent bowel cancer. Based on a 2011 study conducted by the University of Texas MD Anderson Cancer Center, researchers found that the curcumin extract effectively differentiates between cancer cells and normal cells while activating cancer cell death (apoptosis).
Investigators concluded, "Curcumin exerts its biological influence through epigenetic modulation, a process that continues downstream staying one step ahead of adverse genetic influences." (2)

Further, as Dr. Greger wrote concerning another study regarding colon cancer, "...researchers at Cleveland Clinic and John Hopkins School of Medicine tested two phytochemicals, curcumin (from turmeric) and quercitin, (found in fruits and vegetables such as red onions and grapes) in people with familial adenomatous polyposis, an inherited form of colon cancer in which individuals develop hundreds of polyps that may become cancerous unless prophylactically removed."

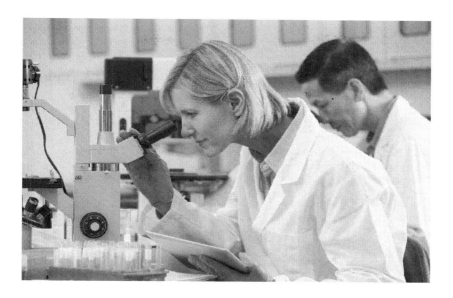

"Researchers gave supplements of curcumin and quercetin to five such patients who already had their colons removed, but still had either polyps in their rectum or in a little intestinal pouch. Each patient had between 5 and 45 polyps each, but after six months on the supplement they ended up with on average fewer than half the polyps, and the ones that were left had shrunk in half. "

"One patient got rid of all polyps by month three, but then they seemed to come back. The researchers asked the patient what's what, and it turned out that the patient stopped taking the supplements. So researchers put the patient back on the phytonutrient supplements for another three months, and the polyps came back down with virtually no adverse events and no blood test abnormalities." (3)

Powerful evidence, among conclusions in many other many studies!

In the West, we recognize the strong anti-inflammatory powers of turmeric and those in the know have been using it in supplements, in food and drinks and even topically. Reducing arthritis, rheumatoid arthritis and inflammatory diseases or the symptoms is of great interest, especially to the aging population that is more prone to develop these diseases.

It is estimated that more than 2 million Americans suffer from rheumatoid arthritis (RA) today and the numbers are increasing. Currently the annual cost of the disease in the US is over $2B. It is typically a progressive degeneration, with much pain and debilitation. Dr. Mercola has treated several thousand RA patients, so he has experience, and he is well-known for digging into alternative and natural treatments.

He says that modern medicine science has not been able to find treatments that significantly improve the long-term outcome of this disease – and the current drugs have nasty side-effects.

He refers to a study that ..."revealed that a highly bioavailable form of curcumin was more effective in alleviating RA symptoms, including tenderness and swelling of joints, than the [NSAID] drug. Not only that, those who were taking the curcumin only, actually experienced the most improvement across the board."

"Along with relieving the most symptoms, the curcumin group [vs the NSAID group] had another benefit – lack of any observed adverse effects. No one in the curcumin group withdrew from the study due to side effects, but 14 percent of those in the NSAID group did so." (4)

There are many studies in this area – suffice it to say that turmeric is an excellent anti-inflammatory. Turmeric is known to help with pain management by using it daily, including for arthritis.

But turmeric helps in other ways.

Dr. Schnaubelt has written that turmeric may have the ability to interfere with cell signaling pathways used in the treatment of squamous cell carcinoma and in melanoma as well as in other cancers. (5)

Oxidative damage is believed to be one of the mechanisms behind aging and many diseases. Turmeric and curcumin are strong anti-oxidants.

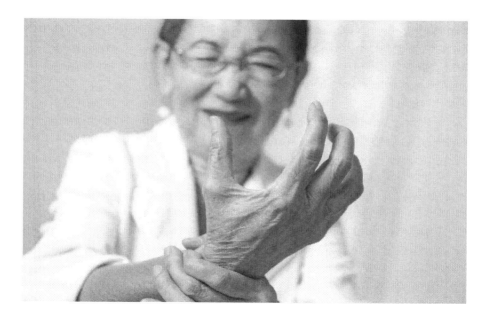

According to UCLA's Neurology Alzheimer center, "Curcumin is recognized by the National Cancer Institute (NCI) and academic investigators around the world as a potent anti-carcinogen. Because of low toxicity and great efficacy in multiple in vitro and in vivo cancer models, curcumin went through extensive toxicology testing and has successively made it through the first stages (Phase I) of clinical testing abroad; it is currently in clinical trials at several sites in the U.S. This work by many labs has provided the basis to quickly and safely explore curcumin's potential for Alzheimer's and other neurological diseases." (7)

It is known that inflammation and oxidative damage play a role in Alzheimer's disease. Curcumin has beneficial effects on both.

The same center says "Curcumin has shown efficacy in many other pre-clinical culture and animal models for diseases related to aging. Treatments with related "curcuminoids" have even been able to increase the lifespan of mice. " (8)

In another study regarding the heart, (8BB) 121 patients who were undergoing coronary artery bypass surgery were randomized to either placebo or 4 grams of curcumin per day, a few days before and after the surgery. The curcumin group had a 65% decreased risk of experiencing a heart attacks.

In summary, while we have only touched on a few research tests to demonstrate different powers of turmeric, understand that it is recognized as an excellent aid for inflammatory diseases, proactive for bowel health, proactive for Alzheimer's or possibly able to slow the disease, is helpful for maintenance of heart health – and more.

There is a link in the reference section pointing to the vast number of scientific and clinical papers on file regarding turmeric and curcumin. (a)

CHAPTER 2

SO WHAT IS TURMERIC?

We have seen some of the benefits of WHY to consider using Turmeric. Now let's look at WHAT it is!

Turmeric is a tropical plant with a bulbous root! To be more exact, it's a rhizomatous herbaceous perennial plant native to Asia. (A rhizome is a root or under-earth thick stem.) Turmeric has an earthy, root-like scent that is subtle and is actually related to ginger. It is a key ingredient in Indian cuisine and other Asian dishes.

It is very high in vitamins and minerals, especially vitamin C. Turmeric's "super power" is Curcumin! Curcumin is the active ingredient in turmeric responsible for the strong anti-inflammatory and antioxidant powers.

Curcumin is the most active constituent of turmeric, making up between 2 % to 6% percent of this spice. The Latin biological name of turmeric is "Curcuma Longa".

Typically turmeric is used in its powder form. That is, the rhizomes are boiled then dried out in an oven, then crushed into powder. The essential oil is extracted through steam distillation or CO_2 distillation.
In some areas, fresh turmeric is used, like ginger.

AS ALLUDED TO IN CHAPTER 1, PROPERTIES OF TURMERIC ARE:

- Analgesic (this means pain relieving)
- Anti-arthritic and anti-inflammatory
- Anti-bacterial
- Digestive aid

- Diuretic (this means to help increase urination)
- Laxative
- Rubefacient (this means it can help with dilation of the capillaries and increase in blood circulation)
- Stimulant, especially immune system stimulant
- Hypotensive (this means lowering blood pressure

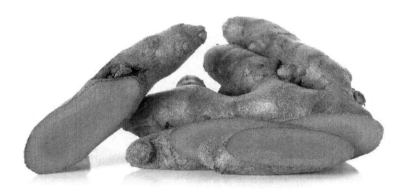

TWO FUN FACTS:

1- In ancient Rome, turmeric was used by the wealthy for wellness, considered a luxury.

2- In medieval Europe, turmeric became known as Indian saffron because it was used widely as an alternative to the far more expensive saffron spice. It was also used as a dye in some areas historically.

_____

In Aromatherapy, turmeric grounds the spirit, helps center scattered or unfocused energy. It warms the body, and can help calm anger and stress.

Turmeric is sold in various forms and found in various products: you can buy the powdered spice for use in cooking and your own recipes (whether for medicinal, skincare or dietary purposes); you can buy supplements; you can find it in soaps & skincare; and there is even an essential oil.

I cooked many Persian dishes and other Middle Eastern dishes when I lived in Paris, and turmeric is almost always in the recipes! It is very much used in India dishes, of course; and it is found in many Asian recipes; In Vietnam, for instance, it's used in countless soups and stir fries. The well- used spice blend, Ras el Hanout in Morocco, typically includes turmeric.

Today I sprinkle it on vegetables, use it in smoothies, drink the tea and sprinkle it in various meat dishes and soups.
I have included a few recipes (from various sources) in the next chapter!

CHAPTER 3

HOW CAN I USE TURMERIC?

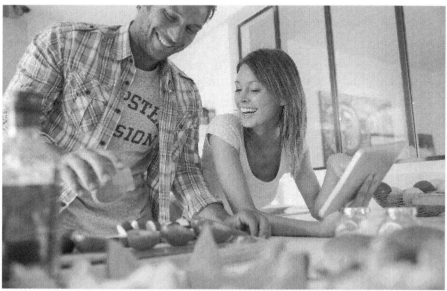

Turmeric can be used in many ways, and easily incorporated into your daily lifestyle, such as:

- ✓ TURMERIC IN COOKING & BAKING
- ✓ TURMERIC IN TEA
- ✓ TURMERIC IN SMOOTHIES & MILK
- ✓ TURMERIC ESSENTIAL OIL
- ✓ TURMERIC ALL-NATURAL SOAP
- ✓ TURMERIC SUPPLEMENTS
- ✓ TURMERIC IN HOME REMEDIES SUCH AS IN COMPRESSES, PASTES FOR WOUNDS, FOR INDIGESTION, FOR SOOTHING STRESS, IN FACIAL MASKS, TO TREAT POST-VIRAL INFECTIONS, IN MASSAGE OILS

Suggested use in foods is about 1 – 1 ½ teaspoons per day, and a typical supplement is about 250 mg per day though those with certain conditions may benefit from 400-500 mg per day with physician or holistic doctor approval.

SEE CAVEATS & CAUTIONS!

<u>TAKE NOTE</u>:

Turmeric is far better absorbed and used by the body when you take it with or include use of Black Pepper, Healthy Fats, Fish Oil, lecithin, an Egg or with a meal.

A research paper found on NIH states: Co- supplementation with 20 mg of piperine (extracted from black pepper) significantly increase the bioavailablity of curcumin by 2000% (9)

Animal studies suggest that curcumin and fish oil synergize very well and improve the results of curcumin & turmeric.

IDEAS & RECIPES!

Turmeric is easy to use in food & drink. Here are just a few ideas followed by some recipes.

A FEW IDEAS

- ✓ ADD SOME TURMERIC TO YOUR SOUPS (I LOVE IT IN BEAN SOUP!)
- ✓ SPRINKLE SOME TURMERIC ON YOUR RICE (ESPECIALLY BASMATI RICE) TO ADD COLOR & BENEFIT
- ✓ MIX SOME TURMERIC INTO YOUR SALAD DRESSING OR OLIVE OIL
- ✓ PUT SOME TURMERIC IN THE SAUTE PAN WITH YOUR ONIONS, GARLIC OR GREENS
- ✓ INCLUDE SOME IN YOUR BREADED SPICES or RUBS FOR BAKED CHICKEN (I USE IT WITH   AN ITALIAN MIX, OREGANO & BREAD CRUMBS)
- ✓ INCLUDE SOME IN YOUR FAVORITE SMOOTHIE
- ✓ PUT ½ TSP IN YOUR BURGER, MEAT LOAF, OR SHREDDED MEAT AND MIX (WE DO THIS   IN KABOBS & MEAT ROLLS)
- ✓ EXCELLENT IN POTATO SALAD!

BE CREATIVE – TRY A LITTLE IN YOUR FAVORITE FOODS OR RECIPES!

A FEW RECIPES

TURMERIC MILK

2 cups of almond milk, coconut milk or any milk of your preference

1 teaspoon of turmeric

¼ teaspoon of black pepper

If you want a little sweetness, add a touch of honey.

Whisk the ingredients together (except honey) then heat in a saucepan until bubble start to show. Remove from heat, stir (and add in honey if you wish). It's ready to sip and drink!

It is equally nice at bedtime as in the day. It helps with digestion, with inflammation, is calming and healthy!

TURMERIC SMOOTHIE

What I love about Smoothies is the creativity
in adding fruits & vegetables.
Here is one fruit recipe to share:

1 cup of coconut milk, almond milk or water
½ to 1 banana

1 tsp chia seeds (or other seeds of your choice)
½ cup of pineapple
½ cup of green melon
1 teaspoon of turmeric

A dash of black pepper

½ teaspoon of ginger (optional)

Note: I like to put peeled perfect bananas in the freezer (in a freeze-
bag) and pull them out as I need them. It helps the smoothie to be
very cold and tasty, and bananas keep longer.

TURMERIC SMOOTHIE II

This one features more vegetables or greens.

1 cup almond or coconut milk or water
1 banana
1 cup fresh baby spinach
¼ cup kale or other greens of choice
½ cup watermelon
½ cup of melon (cantelope or green)
¼ cup pineapple
1 tsp turmeric
Dash of black pepper
Chia, sesame or seeds of choice

TURMERIC TEA

I tend to drink an organic brand of tea mixed with meadowsweet, but here is a recipe I have used:

1 cup water
1 teaspoon turmeric
1 teaspoon cinnamon
¼ teaspoon of clove
Optional – pinch of ginger
½ teaspoon of black pepper
honey to taste

Just bring your water to a boil, stir in the ingredients, let them sit for about 10 minutes, add honey if needed.

SAUCE FOR GREEN BEANS, MEAT OR FISH

GREEN BEANS: Prep your green beans (steam, boil, etc.), set aside.

Melt butter in a saucepan over medium heat, stir in onions, salt & pepper, garlic if you wish, and ½ teaspoon of turmeric. Stir until cooked then mix in green beans. Stir and toss for a minute, be sure the beans are coated.

Remove and eat!

OTHER VEGGIES: You can use a similar process with your favorite greens or other vegetables. I sometimes saute the mix above, and then pour with cold fresh vegetables like radishes, cucumbers, carrots, beans & nuts.

MEAT OR FISH: Use a similar sauce with fish or meats!

There are endless ways to use turmeric in your foods and recipes, and tons of recipe books out there as well. The point is to show you that incorporating turmeric in your foods is an easy and fun way to improve wellness! Be creative and do it!

Now let's turn to some other ways to use turmeric and curcumin in your daily life!

TURMERIC PASTE FOR WOUNDS

Turmeric is a natural disinfectant and can help with wound healing Consider using it in several ways:

Simplest of Pastes: Mix 2 teaspoons of ground turmeric with enough water to make a thick paste (generally about half the amount of turmeric you use). Be sure to wash your hands and then apply the paste gently on the wound. There will be some staining of cloth & skin from this paste.

A More Detailed Paste: Make a paste using turmeric, olive oil, tea tree oil, vitamin E, aloe, beeswax, arnica, and jojoba oil. Apply this formula over the wound for quick relief.

Linseed Paste: Mix some turmeric into linseed oil paste and apply to a wound for pain reduction and to prevent infection.
Use turmeric essential oil in your favorite organic cream or oil, or after a patch test, use a drop "neat" (direct on skin – not typically done) for wound healing. Use 1-2 drops in the paste recipes above.

SOOTHING BATH OR FOOT BATH

Because turmeric is antioxidant, antiseptic and anti-inflammatory, and can help with joint pain, nothing could be more soothing than a turmeric bath! This is a favorite in Japan!

Add ½ cup turmeric, and/or drops of your turmeric essential oil, to your warm bath; less to a foot bath (depending on the size of the bowl); use turmeric soap!

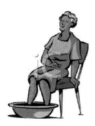

FOR INDIGESTION OR IBS

Blend 6 drops of turmeric essential oil drops into an ounce of oil or cream and massage on your belly.

Using turmeric spice in your food or drinks could help you avoid indigestion.

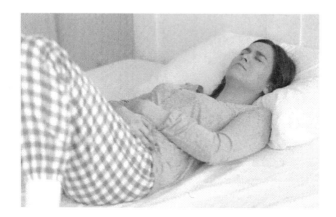

RECOVERY FROM A VIRAL INFECTION

Are you getting over a viral infection or bout?

Turmeric has been shown to help in the recovery from a viral infection. Use turmeric essential oil in a massage, diffuser and/or use it in a soak.

FOR ACNE AND SENSITIVE SKIN

Use turmeric soap for skin with acne, sensitive skin and eczema. The qualities in the soap can help.

For sensitive skin & eczema, you can also put 2-4 drops of turmeric essential oil in an ounce of jojoba and use on skin.

TURMERIC MASK for GLOWING SKIN
Blend together:
1/4 teaspoon turmeric powder
1 teaspoon milk
1 teaspoon honey

Mix, apply to face, let sit for 10 minutes, rinse well.

TURMERIC MASK FOR MOISTURIZING

1/4 teaspoon turmeric powder

1 tablespoon avocado (mashed up well)
1 teaspoon yogurt

Mix together, apply to face, let sit for 10 minutes, rinse well.

CHAPTER 4

ANY CAVEATS?

BLOOD THINNERS ? If you are on blood thinners like Warfarin or Xarelto, avoid excessive use of turmeric and check with your doctor. Turmeric acts as a blood thinner.

BILE DISEASE? If you create excess bile or have a disease regarding bile, check with your doctor first since turmeric steps up bile production.

ABSORPTION. Absorption of curcumin by your body is enhanced with black pepper, ginger and/or fats.

For Better Absorption (specifically for RA or arthritis sufferers), Dr. Mercola suggests:
Make an emulsion by combining a tablespoon of curcumin powder with 1-2 egg yolks and a teaspoon or two of melted coconut oil. Then use a hand blender on high speed to emulsify the powder.

Turmeric/Curcumin is generally recognized as safe (GRAS) on the FDA's GRAS list. The European Food Safety Commission (EU), which has stricter requirements than the FDA for food safety, has also designated curcumin as safe.

CHAPTER 5

An Audio on Turmeric Essential Oil

THIS IS A SHORT AUDIO ABOUT TURMERIC ESSENTIAL OIL:
http://productsonly.libsyn.com/zen-turmeric-essential-oil

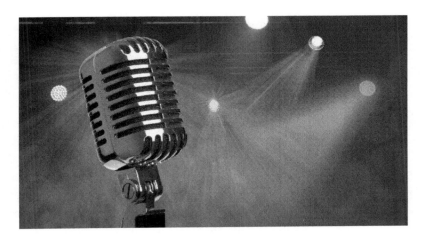

MP3 http://traffic.libsyn.com/productsonly/tumeric.mp3

REFERENCES

a) https://www.ncbi.nlm.nih.gov/pubmed/?term=curcumin

1)   http://www.ncbi.nlm.nih.gov/pubmed/24513290
http://www.ncbi.nlm.nih.gov/pubmed/25159739
http://www.ncbi.nlm.nih.gov/pubmed/25173461

2)   https://thetruthaboutcancer.com/benefits-turmeric-cancer-treatment/

3)   Dr. Greger http://nutritionfacts.org/2015/10/22/preventing-and-treating-colon-cancer-with-turmeric-curcumin/

4)   Dr. Mercola
http://articles.mercola.com/sites/articles/archive/2012/06/13/the-spice-that-is-better-than-drugs-for-ra.aspx

5)   Dr. Schnaubelt "The Healing Intelligence of Essential Oils". Healing Arts Press. 2011. pg 162.
6)   IBID

7)   http://alzheimer.neurology.ucla.edu/Curcumin.html

8)   IBID

9)   https://www.ncbi.nlm.nih.gov/pubmed/22481014

10) Pepper and bioavailability
https://www.ncbi.nlm.nih.gov/pmc/articles/PMC2781139/

⍰

ABOUT THE AUTHOR

Kathy Heshelow is an Amazon best-selling author, and has written a number of books over the years. She is starting a frequent series of book in 2017 on wellness subjects.

Her two areas of focus are wellness / beauty; and passive income real estate investing with the 1031 tax deferred strategy. She runs a skincare line (Sublime Beauty), a wellness company (Sublime Naturals) and ZEN BOX, an essential oil subscription box.

She actually learned many of the wellness skills and concepts when she lived in Paris, France for 16 years (such as Skin Brushing, Essential Oils for wellness, European skin care techniques.) This has prompted her to start the Sublime Wellness Lifestyle Series of eBooks, with the book on Turmeric appearing first.

Previously published:
 "Essential Oils Have Super Powers: from Solving Everyday Wellness Problems to Taking on Super Bugs" + the Series
"The Crisis of Antibiotic-Resistant Bacteria and How Essential Oils Can Help"
"Mind Body Spirit and Aromatherapy"
"Anecdotes, Fun Facts & Fascinating History of Essential Oils"
"Phytoceramides: Anti Aging at its Best"
"Secrets to a Better Immune System"
"Turmeric: How to Use it For Your Wellness"
"Secrets to a Stronger Immune System"

Passive Real Estate Investing on Amazon
NNN – 1031 Defer Taxes and Gain Passive Income in Commercial Real Estate
The ABCs of TICs
The ABCs of DPPs

She has a new podcast on iTunes, "Essential Oil Zen".

Join Kathy's list to get free promos, early copies and news on new books.

Join at www.kathyheshelow.com

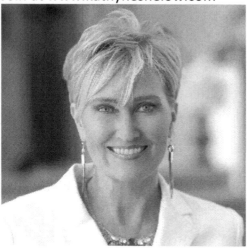

IF YOU NEED HELP TO GET STARTED WITH TURMERIC:

TURMERIC LOVERS GIFT BOX
found on SublimeNaturals.com

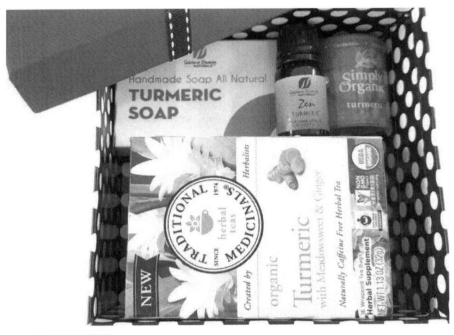

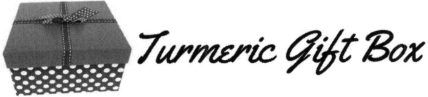

AVAILABLE ON AMAZON AND ON SUBLIMENATURALS.COM

TURMERIC ESSENTIAL OIL

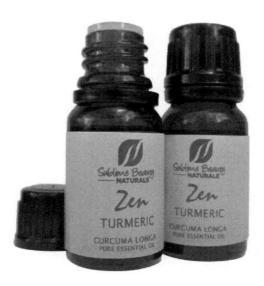

Available on Amazon or SublimeNaturals.com

TURMERIC NATURAL HANDMADE SOAP

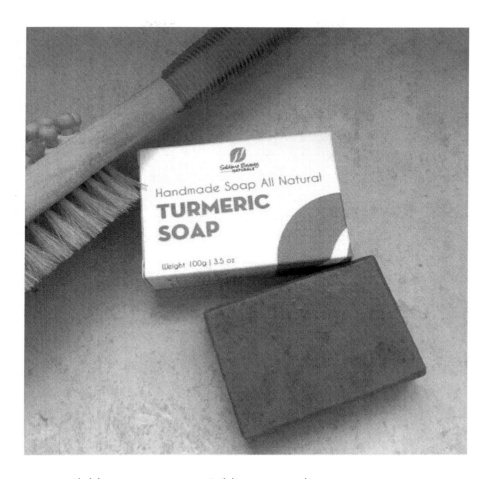

Available on Amazon or SublimeNaturals.com

I hope you have enjoyed this short journey with Turmeric and Curcumin.

I'd love to hear from you if you have questions.

Do leave a review on Amazon about the book.

Warmly, Kathy Heshelow

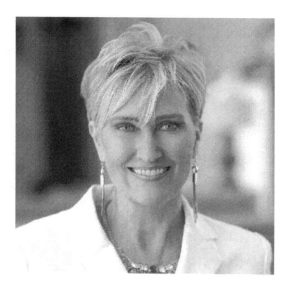

Made in the USA
Columbia, SC
16 February 2019